Evaluation of Knowledge, Attitudes, and Practices Regarding Influenza Vaccination Among Employees in a School District

Marie A. de Perio, MD
Douglas M. Wiegand, PhD
Scott E. Brueck, MS, CIH

HHE | HealthHazard Evaluation Program

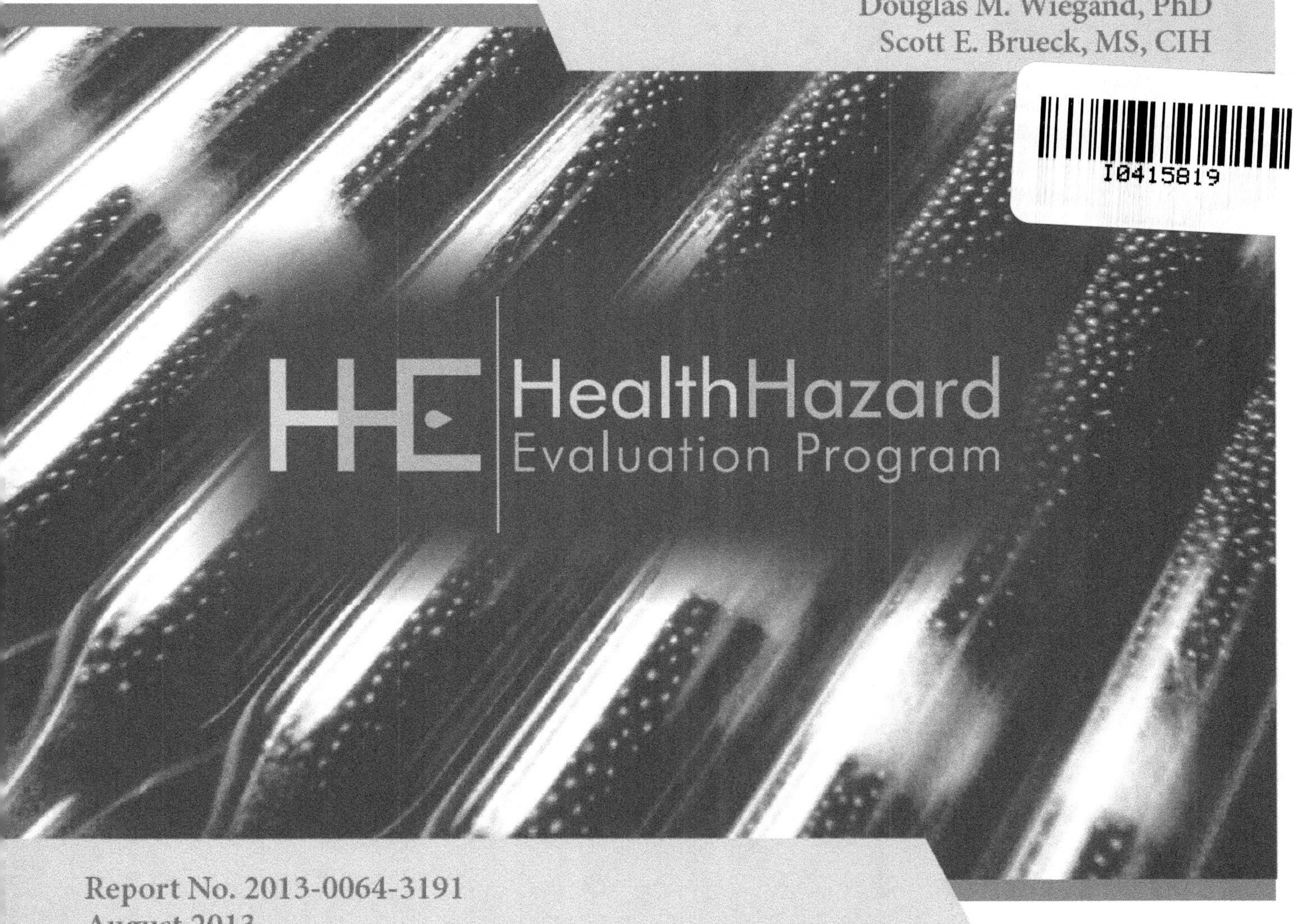

Report No. 2013-0064-3191
August 2013

U.S. Department of Health and Human Services
Centers for Disease Control and Prevention
National Institute for Occupational Safety and Health

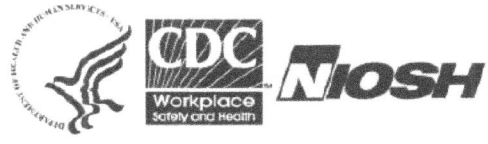

Contents

The employer is required to post a copy of this report for 30 days at or near the workplace(s) of affected employees. The employer must take steps to ensure that the posted report is not altered, defaced, or covered by other material.

The cover photo is a close-up image of sorbent tubes, which are used by the HHE Program to measure airborne exposures. This photo is an artistic representation that may not be related to this Health Hazard Evaluation.

Highlights of this Evaluation

The Health Hazard Evaluation Program received a request from a management representative at a school district. The request asked for our assistance in examining influenza vaccination (flu vaccine) coverage among school district employees. The request also asked for assistance in assessing attitudes and beliefs toward the vaccine. Vaccination is the most effective method to prevent influenza and to prevent serious illness and death from influenza infection.

What We Did

- We surveyed 412 (49%) of the 841 employees at the school district using a web-based questionnaire in March 2013.

- We asked employees what they knew and thought about the flu vaccine.

- We asked employees whether they had received the flu vaccine.

What We Found

- Fifty-eight percent of responding school district employees reported getting the flu vaccine for the 2012–2013 season. Most reported getting it at the central district office.

- The most common reasons for not getting the vaccine were beliefs that employees did not need the vaccine, that the vaccine did not work, and that employees did not have time to get it.

- Employees with positive attitudes and perceptions about the flu vaccine and those who received the vaccine the previous year were more likely to have been vaccinated.

> We examined the knowledge, attitudes, beliefs, and receipt of the influenza vaccine among 412 school district employees. We found influenza vaccination coverage to be 58% in our respondents. The most common reasons for not getting the vaccine included believing that the vaccine was not needed, that the vaccine did not work, and that employees did not have time to get vaccinated. Future vaccination campaigns should emphasize the benefits, safety, and effectiveness of vaccination.

What the Employer Can Do

- Work with local vaccine providers to offer the flu vaccine to employees at each of the schools.

- Educate employees about the flu and the flu vaccine. Focus on their risk of infection and the effectiveness and safety of the vaccine.

What Employees Can Do

- Get the flu vaccine every year. Vaccination is the most effective way to avoid getting the flu, which can cause lost time from work, serious illness, and death.

- Stay informed. Get information about the flu and the flu vaccine from reliable sources.

- Do not go to work when ill with flu-like symptoms, which can include fever, cough, and sore throat.

Mention of any company or product does not constitute endorsement by NIOSH. In addition, citations to websites external to NIOSH do not constitute NIOSH endorsement of the sponsoring organizations or their programs or products. Furthermore, NIOSH is not responsible for the content of these websites. All web addresses referenced in this document were accessible as of the publication date of this report.

Abbreviations

ACIP   Advisory Committee on Immunization Practices
AOR   Adjusted odds ratio
CI   Confidence interval
ILI   Influenza-like illness
NIOSH   National Institute for Occupational Safety and Health
OR   Odds ratio

Introduction

The Health Hazard Evaluation Program received a request from the director of human resources at a school district. The request asked for our assistance in examining influenza vaccination coverage among school district employees. We used a web-based survey to determine influenza vaccination coverage among school employees in the district. We also assessed knowledge and attitudes toward vaccination and the prevalence of influenza-like illness (ILI) symptoms.

School District

At the time of our evaluation, the school district was a comprehensive preschool through 12th grade school district in the suburbs of a large city in Ohio. The district had five elementary schools, one middle school, and two high schools and served nearly 7,800 students. It had 841 full-time and part-time employees, including 444 teachers, 93 paraprofessionals and aides, 21 principals and assistant principals, 44 administrative assistants, 22 counselors and therapists, 5 psychologists, 4 school nurses, 49 food services workers, 46 maintenance and custodial workers, and 65 bus drivers and monitors.

The school district had offered employees influenza vaccination at the central district administration office every year for at least 17 years. For the 2012–2013 influenza season, the influenza vaccine was offered in injection form to employees at the central district office one afternoon (1:00 p.m.–5:30 p.m.) in October 2012. The central district office is in a building next to one of the high schools. The school district notified employees of the opportunity to receive the influenza vaccine by e-mail and posted flyers. Employees covered under the school district's health insurance plan obtained the vaccine free of charge. Employees not covered under this plan obtained the vaccine for $25.99. According to the school district nurse, 202 employees received the vaccine at the district office on this date.

The district's insurance plan also covered influenza vaccination at physicians' offices and many of the major retail pharmacy chains in the area. The school district had no information on how many employees received the influenza vaccination at these locations.

Influenza

Influenza is a contagious respiratory illness caused by influenza viruses that infect the nose, throat, and lungs. It can cause mild to severe illness and can lead to death. Symptoms of influenza infection include fever, cough, sore throat, runny or stuffy nose, body aches, headache, chills, and fatigue. Some people have vomiting and diarrhea, while others have respiratory symptoms without a fever [CDC 2012c].

Influenza viruses are thought to be spread mainly by droplets made when people with influenza cough, sneeze, or talk. Less often, people might also get influenza by touching a surface or object that has influenza virus on it and then touching their own mouth, eyes, or nose [Wright and Webster 2001]. Evidence for airborne transmission (or aerosolization of small particles that remain suspended in air for long periods) also exists [Bridges et al. 2003; Blachere et al. 2009; Lindsley et al. 2010a,b].

Complications of influenza include bacterial pneumonia, ear infections, sinus infections, dehydration, and worsening of chronic medical conditions [CDC 2012c]. Individuals at higher risk for developing influenza-related complications include children younger than 5 years (especially children younger than 2 years), adults 65 years of age and older, pregnant women, and people with chronic medical conditions (asthma; chronic lung disease; neurological conditions; heart disease; blood, endocrine, kidney, liver, and metabolic disorders; weakened immune system due to human immunodeficiency virus, cancer, or medication; and morbid obesity) [CDC 2012c]. Obesity, defined as a body mass index ≥ 30, has also recently been shown to be associated with influenza-related complications [CDC 2009b; Jain et al. 2009; Kumar et al. 2009; Louie et al. 2009; Kwong et al. 2011].

In the United States, more than 200,000 people each year are hospitalized for influenza-related illnesses [Thompson et al. 2004]. CDC estimates that from 1976 to 2007, influenza-associated deaths ranged from a low of about 3,000 to a high of about 49,000 people per year in the United States [CDC 2010a]. Influenza has been estimated to cause more than 70 million lost working days and $6.2 billion in lost productivity in the United States each year [Adams et al. 1999; Molinari et al. 2007].

Influenza Vaccines

Vaccination is the most effective method to prevent influenza and to prevent serious illness and death from influenza infection [Cox and Subbarao 1999; Nichol and Treanor 2006]. The 2012–2013 seasonal influenza vaccine for the U.S. population became available in August 2012. The U.S. influenza vaccines contained the A/California/7/2009 (H1N1)-like, A/Victoria/361/2011 (H3N2)-like, and B/Wisconsin/1/2010-like (Yamagata lineage) antigens [CDC 2012d].

In 2010, the Advisory Committee on Immunization Practices (ACIP) first recommended annual influenza vaccination for all persons aged ≥ 6 months in the United States [CDC 2010b]. ACIP continued to recommend annual influenza vaccination for all persons aged ≥ 6 months for the 2012–2013 season [CDC 2012d].

The efficacy of influenza vaccines in adults has been shown to be 70%–90% against confirmed influenza when the vaccine strains match the circulating strains [Fukuda et al. 2004]. Influenza vaccination has also been shown to reduce the rates of ILI, lost workdays, and physician visits in healthy, working adults when the vaccine and circulating viruses are similar [Nichol et al. 1995; Bridges et al. 2000]. The interim estimate of overall influenza vaccine effectiveness for preventing laboratory-confirmed influenza virus infection associated with medically attended acute respiratory infection for the 2012–2013 influenza season was determined to be 56% (95% confidence interval [CI] = 47%–63%) [CDC 2013b]. Vaccine effectiveness was estimated as 47% against influenza A (H3N2) virus infections and 67% against B virus infections [CDC 2013b].

The inactivated influenza injection vaccine contains inactivated viruses and cannot cause influenza in people who get the vaccine [CDC 2010b]. The most common side effect of seasonal influenza injection vaccines reported in adults is soreness at the injection site [Vellozzi et al. 2009]. Muscle pain, discomfort or weakness, and fever rarely occur. The live attenuated influenza nasal vaccine contains a weakened virus and cannot cause influenza in those who get the vaccine. However, it can cause mild signs or symptoms including runny nose, nasal congestion, fever, or sore throat. These side effects are mild and short-lasting, especially when compared to the symptoms of seasonal influenza infection [CDC 2010b].

In the United States, approximately 55 million students and 7 million staff attend more than 130,000 public and private schools each day. School settings place teachers and other school employees at risk for influenza infection and subsequent transmission to others. Schools have the potential to become centers of influenza outbreaks because of their large population, high levels of close social contact, and interaction with the community [Gargano et al. 2011]. Vaccinating this group could help protect one fifth of the country's population from influenza [CDC 2012a].

Healthy People 2020, a national health promotion and disease prevention initiative, sets the target seasonal influenza vaccination coverage rate for non-institutionalized high-risk adults aged 18 to 64 years at 80% [U.S. Department of Health and Human Services 2013]. Data regarding seasonal influenza vaccination rates among teachers and other school employees is limited. In the only published study on this topic, Gargano and colleagues found that 62% of 66 surveyed school employees received the 2009–2010 seasonal influenza vaccine in two rural counties in Georgia. This study focused on teachers and staff at middle and high schools. Employees with higher perceived severity of influenza infection in general and increased comfort in getting the influenza vaccination were more likely to have received the influenza vaccine [Gargano et al. 2011]. Information on knowledge and attitudes toward seasonal influenza vaccination among all types of school employees in non-rural areas is lacking.

Methods

The purpose of our evaluation was to (1) determine 2012–2013 influenza vaccination coverage rates among employees in the school district, (2) assess employees' knowledge and attitudes toward vaccination, (3) determine factors associated with acceptance and refusal of the vaccine, (4) determine the prevalence of ILI among employees, and (5) provide recommendations to the school district to improve influenza vaccination campaigns for their employees.

Survey Design

We surveyed school district employees to examine their knowledge, attitudes, and receipt of the influenza vaccine. The study population for this evaluation consisted of all 841 paid employees. All part-time and full-time employees ≥ 18 years old, including educational, administrative, and operational staff, were invited to participate. We communicated with the director of human resources, the district nurse, and the leaders of the two unions (representing paraprofessionals/aides and operation employees) and the teachers' association in planning and carrying out the survey.

We used the Theory of Planned Behavior, a widely accepted theory in predicting social and health behavior, in developing the questionnaire [Ajzen 1991; Armitage and Conner 2001]. The Theory of Planned Behavior states that a person's attitude (positive or negative feelings toward a behavior), perception of subjective norms (the perception that there is social pressure to perform or not perform the behavior), and perceived behavioral control (the perception of choice and availability of resources necessary to perform or not perform the behavior) influence a person's intention to perform the behavior. When a person has a positive attitude toward a behavior and feels that others encourage the behavior, and he or she has the choice and resources to perform the behavior, then intention to perform the behavior will typically be positive. Survey items measured attitudes towards the vaccine, subjective norms regarding receiving the vaccine, and perceived behavioral control in receiving the vaccine [Francis et al. 2004; de Perio et al. 2012].

Some knowledge and attitudes questions were examined by extent of agreement with statements about each vaccine, using a four-point Likert scale (i.e., disagree, somewhat disagree, somewhat agree, agree). Other attitudes questions were examined using a four-point scale with bipolar adjectives (e.g., very good, somewhat good, somewhat bad, very bad).

The survey also included questions regarding participant demographics, work history, pertinent medical history, receipt of the influenza vaccine, and ILI symptoms since the start of the school year. Demographic questions from the Behavioral Risk Factor Surveillance System Survey Questionnaire [CDC 2011a] and influenza vaccine practices questions adapted from the National 2009 H1N1 Flu Survey Questionnaire were used [CDC 2009a]. The questionnaire was reviewed by subject matter experts from CDC's Immunization Services Division. The questionnaire included no personal identifying information such as names or dates of birth.

At the school district's request, the survey was Web-based because all district employees had an e-mail address and access to the Web. We used the survey tool in the EpiInfo™ 7 Publish Form to Web Service. An information sheet was distributed 2 weeks before survey launch to the union and teachers' association leaders and the district's director of human resources for dissemination to each school. The survey was available over a 3-week period from March 5–26, 2013. The survey link was sent to all school district employees by the director of human resources with multiple reminders given over the 3 weeks. Only National Institute for Occupational Safety and Health (NIOSH) investigators had access to the survey data.

Data Analysis

Survey results were analyzed by using descriptive statistical methods such as frequencies, proportions, means, and standard deviations as appropriate. Responses that used a Likert scale were categorized as "expressed agreement" if respondents marked "agree" or "somewhat agree," and as "expressed disagreement" if respondents marked "disagree" or "somewhat disagree." Internal consistency for the attitudes, subjective norms, and perceived behavioral control variables was analyzed using Cronbach's coefficient (α) after adjusting for the directionality of items, where necessary. We created composite scores for variables within the attitudes, subjective norms, and perceived behavioral control domains where $\alpha > 0.6$ by calculating the mean of the individual scores for each respondent.

Characteristics of school employees who reported receipt of the influenza vaccine were compared to those who denied receipt of the vaccine. Responses to the knowledge and attitudes questions were compared among each group. In addition, characteristics of school employees who reported ILI symptoms were compared to those who denied ILI symptoms. ILI was defined as being sick with fever and either sore throat or cough at any time from August 22, 2012, through survey completion.

Bivariate analyses used the Student's t-test, $\chi 2$ test, or Fisher's exact test. We used logistic regression for the bivariate analyses of the composite scores for the attitudes, subjective norms, and perceived behavioral control domains. Associations were expressed as odds ratios (OR) with their 95% confidence intervals. The OR is an estimate of relative risk, which is calculated by comparing the odds of some outcome (e.g., receipt of vaccine versus non-receipt of vaccine) occurring given the presence of some predictor factor, condition, or classification (e.g., male versus female). It is usually a comparison of the presence of a condition to its absence (e.g., receipt of vaccine and non-receipt of vaccine). An OR of 1.0 indicates that the outcome is equally likely to occur given the condition. An OR greater than 1.0 indicates that the outcome is more likely to occur given the condition. ORs of less than 1.0 indicate that the outcome is less likely to occur [Pedhazur 1997]. The ORs presented in this report are accompanied by a lower confidence level and upper confidence level. An OR is considered statistically significant if the confidence level range does not include 1.0.

All tests were two-tailed, and statistical significance was set at $P < 0.05$. We then used a multiple logistic regression model to identify factors independently associated with receipt of the vaccine. All analyses were conducted using CDC EpiInfo 7.1.1.0 with the exception of calculation of the Cronbach's α, which used IBM SPSS Statistics Predictive Analytics Software version 18.0.

Results

Demographic and Health Characteristics of Survey Respondents

A total of 412 (49%) of 841 employees completed a survey. The median age of the respondents was 46 years, with a range of 22–71 years. Most (82%) of respondents were female. Most (99%) respondents self-identified their race as white. Other demographic characteristics of survey respondents are shown in Table 1.

Table 1. Demographic characteristics of survey respondents

Demographic characteristic	No. (%) respondents n = 399–412*
Female	337 (82)
Pregnant at the time of survey completion	7 (2)
White race	406 (99)
Hispanic ethnicity	2 (0.5)
Highest year of school completed	
Some college or technical school or less	78 (19)
College graduate or more	330 (81)
Annual household income	
< $35,000	16 (4)
≥ $35,000	383 (96)
Household included:	
One or more adults ≥ 18 years old†	378 (92)
One or more children ≤ 5 months old	6 (1)
One or more children 6 months–17 years old	193 (47)

*Sample sizes ranged from 399–412 because of missing values.

†Respondents were asked to exclude themselves when answering this question.

Regarding current underlying medical conditions, 21 (5%) reported having asthma; 3 (1%) reported having another lung disease; 11 (3%) reported having diabetes mellitus; 9 (2%) reported having heart disease; and 14 (4%) reported having a weakened immune system caused by active cancer, a chronic illness, or by medicines taken for a chronic illness. In total, 345 (88%) of the 394 respondents who reported this information denied having a medical condition placing them at higher risk for influenza complications. We calculated body mass index for each participant on the basis of their self-reported height and weight using the following formula:

$$\text{weight (pounds)} / \text{height (inches)}^2 \times 703$$

Of 386 respondents, 73 (19%) were classified as obese, which was defined as a body mass index ≥ 30 [CDC 2011b]. Regarding current mental health conditions, 28 (7%) reported having depression and 41 (10%) reported having anxiety. In total, 342 (86%) of 398 respondents indicated that they did not have either condition. We did not ask about other mental health conditions.

Work Characteristics of Survey Respondents

Most (92%) respondents were employed full time by the school district. The median years worked in any school system was 15 years, with a range of 0–44 years. The median years worked in the current school system was 7 years, with a range of 0–41 years. Other work characteristics, including primary occupation and primary workplace, are shown in Table 2.

Table 2. Work characteristics of survey respondents

Work characteristic	No. (%) respondents n = 412
Full time employment	378 (92)
Primary occupation	
Teacher/substitute teacher	250 (61)
Aide/paraprofessional	59 (14)
Administrative assistant	27 (7)
Principal/assistant principal	15 (4)
Bus driver/monitor	14 (3)
Counselor/therapist	12 (3)
Maintenance/custodial worker	8 (2)
Food services worker	6 (1)
Nurse	3 (1)
Other*	18 (4)
Primary workplace	
Elementary school	186 (45)
High school	125 (30)
Middle school	59 (14)
Central district office	21 (5)
Transportation department	17 (4)
Maintenance building	4 (1)

*Other primary occupations included administrator, health aide, librarian, and psychologist.

Response rates for these occupational groups were 75% (3 of 4) for nurses, 71% (15 of 21) for principals/assistant principals, 63% (59 of 93) for aides/paraprofessionals, 56% (250 of 444) for teachers/substitute teachers, 55% (12 of 22) for counselor/therapists, 22% (14 of 65) for bus drivers/monitors, 17% (8 of 46) for maintenance/custodial workers, and 12% (6 of 49) for food services workers.

Influenza Vaccine Receipt, Beliefs, and Attitudes

A total of 245 (60%) of 411 respondents reported getting the 2011–2012 influenza vaccine last season. A total of 238 (58%) of 410 respondents reported getting the 2012–2013 influenza vaccine this season. The cumulative number of respondents receiving the influenza vaccine for the 2012–2013 season by month is shown in Figure 1. Of the respondents who received the influenza vaccine, 68% received it by November 2012. The most common places where respondents received the influenza vaccine were the central district office (58%), a doctor's office (15%), and a pharmacy or drug store (15%). Twelve percent of employees received the vaccine in other locations (hospital, other clinic, supermarket, other nonmedical place).

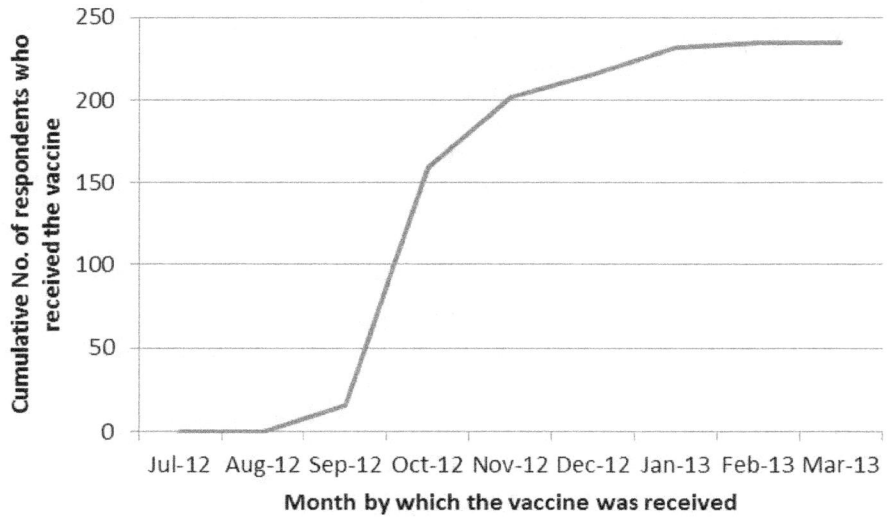

Figure 1. Month when influenza vaccine was received by respondents.

Vaccination rates for the two most common occupational groups were 55% for teachers and 64% for aides/paraprofessionals. Vaccination rates for the other occupational groups ranged from 25%–83% and are shown in Figure 2. In addition, 60% of respondents who reported an underlying high-risk medical condition and 59% of respondents classified as obese reported having received the influenza vaccine.

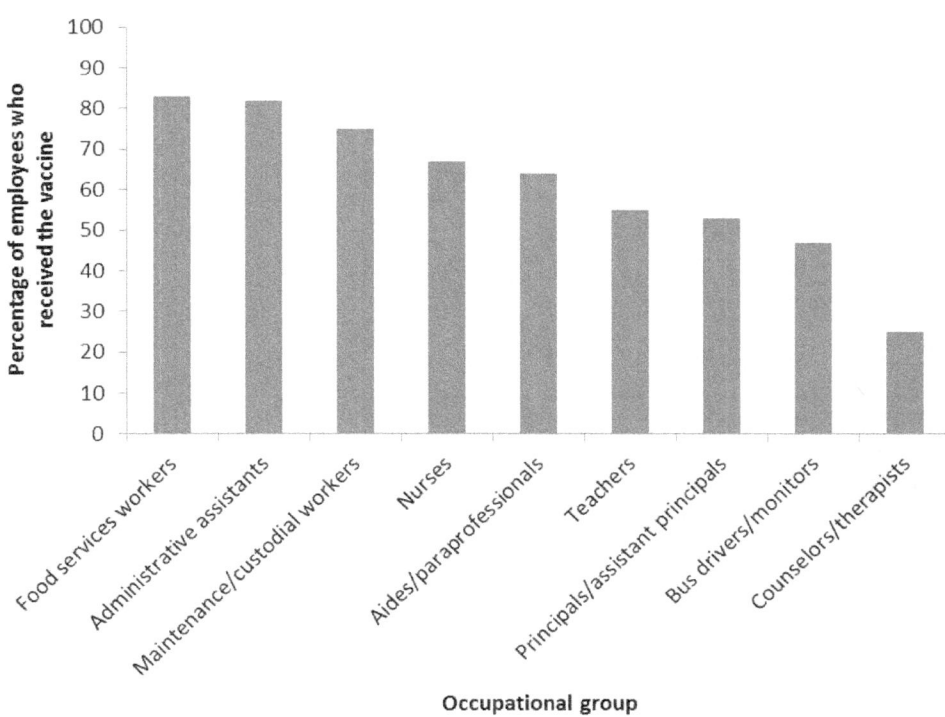

Figure 2. Vaccination coverage by occupational group.

Of the 238 respondents who reported receiving the influenza vaccine, the most common reason for receiving it was to protect oneself or one's family (87%). Other reasons are shown in Table 3.

Table 3. Main reasons cited by respondents who received the flu vaccine

Main reason cited*	No. (%) respondents n = 238
To protect myself/my family	206 (87)
I've read or heard that getting the flu vaccine is recommended	11 (5)
My doctor recommended that I get the flu vaccine	9 (4)
Other	12 (5)

*Respondents were asked to choose one main reason.

Of the 172 respondents who had not received the influenza vaccine, the most common reason cited for not receiving it was "I don't think I need the vaccine" (32%). The next most common reasons were "I don't think the flu vaccine will keep me from getting the flu" (21%) and "I haven't had time to get the flu vaccine" (17%). Other reasons are shown in Table 4.

Table 4. Main reasons cited by respondents for not receiving the flu vaccine

Main reason cited*	No. (%) respondents n = 172
I don't think I need the vaccine.	55 (32)
I don't think the flu vaccine will keep me from getting the flu.	36 (21)
I haven't had time to get the flu vaccine.	29 (17)
I don't think the flu vaccine is safe.	18 (11)
Other†	34 (20)

*Respondents were asked to choose one main reason.

†The most common "other" reasons cited included "I never get the flu" and "I got very sick from a previous flu vaccine."

Most respondents had positive attitudes toward the vaccine, as most believed the vaccine to be "beneficial" (91%), "good" (92%), and "wise" (92%) versus "harmful," "bad," and "unwise." The three positive measures had a Cronbach's (or internal consistency) coefficient of $\alpha = 0.83$. Thus, for subsequent analyses, we created one positive attitudes composite score by calculating the mean of the scores for the three items.

Beliefs about the influenza vaccine are shown in Table 5. Nearly all respondents believed transmission of influenza could occur between teachers/staff and children (99%) and that influenza was a serious infection (96%). Regarding the influenza vaccine, 72% believed the flu vaccine would prevent them from getting the flu. However, most (59%) believed it could make them sick.

Table 5. Beliefs of respondents about the flu vaccine

Belief statement	No. (%) respondents who expressed agreement with statement regarding influenza n = 408–412*
Teachers/staff and children can spread flu amongst each other.	409 (99)
The flu is a serious infection.	392 (96)
The flu vaccine will prevent me from getting the flu.	296 (72)
The flu vaccine could make me sick.	243 (59)

*Sample sizes varied because of missing values.

Respondents' agreement with the subjective norm statements about the influenza vaccine is shown in Table 6. Approximately one third of respondents believed it was their duty to get the vaccine for their job. Between 52%–67% of respondents reported that their manager, doctor, or family/friends wanted them to get the vaccine, while fewer (16%) reported feeling social pressure to get the vaccine. These seven subjective norms items had a Cronbach's coefficient of $\alpha = 0.72$. Thus, for subsequent analyses, we created one subjective norms composite score by calculating the mean of the scores for the seven items.

Table 6. Agreement with subjective norm statements about the influenza vaccine

Subjective norm statement	No. (%) respondents who expressed agreement with statement regarding influenza n = 405–412*
My doctor recommended that I get the flu vaccine.	276 (67)
A majority of my coworkers have gotten or plan to get the vaccine.	227 (55)†
My manager/employer wanted me to get the flu vaccine.	223 (54)
My family/friends wanted me to get the flu vaccine.	221 (55)
People who are important to me wanted me to get the flu vaccine.	216 (52)
It was my duty to get the flu vaccine for my job.	149 (36)
I felt social pressure to get the flu vaccine.	67 (17)

*Sample sizes varied because of missing values.

†For this statement, respondents could also answer "I don't know," and 150 respondents chose this option.

Respondents' agreement with the perceived behavioral control statements about the influenza vaccine is shown in Table 7. Almost all (99%) respondents felt that it was their decision whether or not to get the vaccine. Few respondents felt they did not have the time or money to get the vaccine, and only 11% of respondents felt that getting the vaccine required a lot of effort. The latter three perceived behavioral control items had a Cronbach's coefficient of $\alpha = 0.64$. Thus, for subsequent analyses, we created one perceived behavioral control composite score for each vaccine by calculating the mean of the scores for the three items.

Table 7. Agreement with perceived behavioral control statements about the influenza vaccine

Perceived behavioral control statement	No. (%) respondents who expressed agreement with statement regarding influenza n = 409–412*
It was my decision whether or not to get the flu vaccine.	406 (99)
I did not have time to get the flu vaccine.	67 (16)
I did not have the money to get the flu vaccine.	18 (4)
Getting the flu vaccine required a lot of effort on my part.	47 (11)

*Sample sizes varied because of missing values.

Factors Associated with Influenza Vaccine Receipt

We found no statistically significant associations between sex, race, ethnicity, or highest education level and reporting receipt of the influenza vaccine. However, respondents aged ≥ 50 years were 2.04 times more likely (95% CI = 1.34, 3.11) to have received the influenza vaccine than those aged < 50 years. Neither annual household income nor whether a respondent's household included adults, children, or infants were significantly associated with receipt of the vaccine. Pregnancy, obesity, and having an underlying high-risk medical condition, anxiety, or depression were not significantly associated with receipt of the vaccine.

The mean number of years worked in the school district or in any school system was not significantly associated with receipt of the vaccine. Also, occupation and full-time status were not significantly associated with receipt of the vaccine. However, respondents with a primary workplace at the central district office, where the vaccine was administered, were 3.23 times more likely (95% CI = 1.07, 9.78) to have received the influenza vaccine than those worked at other locations.

Respondents who reported receiving the 2011–2012 influenza vaccine were 36.82 times more likely (95% CI = 20.97, 64.68) to have received the 2012–2013 influenza vaccine compared to those who did not). Respondents who believed in the efficacy of the influenza vaccine were 5.41 times more likely (95% CI = 3.36, 8.70) to have received the vaccine than those who did not believe. Respondents who believed that the vaccine could make them sick were 4 times less likely (95% CI = 0.16, 0.39) to have received the vaccine than those who did not. Expressing agreement with the other belief statements in Table 5 was not significantly associated with receipt of the influenza vaccine.

Respondents with a higher positive attitudes composite score for the influenza vaccine, or those who had more positive attitudes toward the vaccines were 21.46 times more likely (95% CI = 10.97, 41.98) to have received the vaccine. Respondents with a higher subjective norms composite score for the influenza vaccine, or those who felt external pressure from others to receive the vaccine, were 5.99 times more likely (95% CI = 4.10, 8.75) to have received that vaccine. In addition, respondents with a higher perceived behavioral control composite score for the influenza vaccine or those who felt personal control over whether or not to get the vaccine were 4.81 times more likely (95% CI = 3.04, 7.62) to have received that vaccine.

Variables with $P < 0.05$ that were associated with receipt of the 2012–2013 influenza vaccine (except for receipt of the 2011–2012 influenza vaccine) were entered into a multiple logistic regression model to determine which ones were independently associated with receipt of the vaccine (reported as adjusted odds ratios [AOR] in Table 8). Factors independently associated with receipt of the 2012–2013 influenza vaccine included having positive attitudes toward the vaccine (AOR = 12.04, CI = 5.26, 27.56), feeling external pressure to get it (AOR = 4.16, 95% CI = 2.54, 6.83), and feeling personal control over whether or not to get it (AOR = 7.86, 95% CI = 4.07, 15.20). Believing that the vaccine could make them sick was independently associated with not receiving the vaccine (AOR = 0.49, CI = 0.25, 0.94).

Table 8. Logistic regression model for receipt of the 2012–2013 influenza vaccine

Variable	No. (%) received influenza vaccine n = 409–410*	Crude odds ratio (95% CI)	Adjusted odds ratio (95% CI)
Age			
≥ 50 years	105 (68)	2.04 (1.34, 3.11)†	1.28 (0.66, 2.50)
< 50 years	125 (51)		
Primary workplace			
Central district office	17 (81)	3.23 (1.07, 9.78)†	2.85 (0.58, 13.94)
Other location‡	221 (57)		
The flu vaccine will prevent me from getting the flu.			
Agree	203 (69)	5.41 (3.36, 8.70)†	1.98 (0.99, 3.97)
Disagree	33 (29)		
The flu vaccine could make me sick.			
Agree	109 (45)	0.25 (0.16, 0.39)†	0.49 (0.25, 0.94)†
Disagree	128 (77)		
Positive attitudes composite score (i.e., having positive attitudes toward the vaccine)	NA	21.46 (10.97, 41.98)†	12.04 (5.26, 27.56)†
Subjective norms composite score (i.e., feeling external pressure to get the vaccine)	NA	5.99 (4.10, 8.75)†	4.16 (2.54, 6.83)†
Perceived behavioral control composite score (i.e., feeling personal control over whether or not to get the vaccine)	NA	4.81 (3.04, 7.62)†	7.86 (4.07, 15.20)†

*Sample sizes varied because of missing values.
†$P < 0.05$
‡Other primary workplace included school, transportation department, or maintenance building.

Influenza-like Illness

A total of 120 (29%) responding employees reported ILI symptoms from August 22, 2012, through survey completion. The month of illness onset is shown in Figure 3. A peak in illness occurred in January 2013 when 28 respondents reported onset of their ILI symptoms. Sixty-eight (57%) respondents who reported ILI symptoms also reported receiving the influenza vaccine. However, 8 (14%) of these respondents reported their ILI symptoms before receiving their influenza vaccine.

Four (3%) respondents reporting ILI symptoms reported an influenza diagnosis via a nasopharyngeal swab. None of these four respondents reported having received the 2012–2013 influenza vaccine.

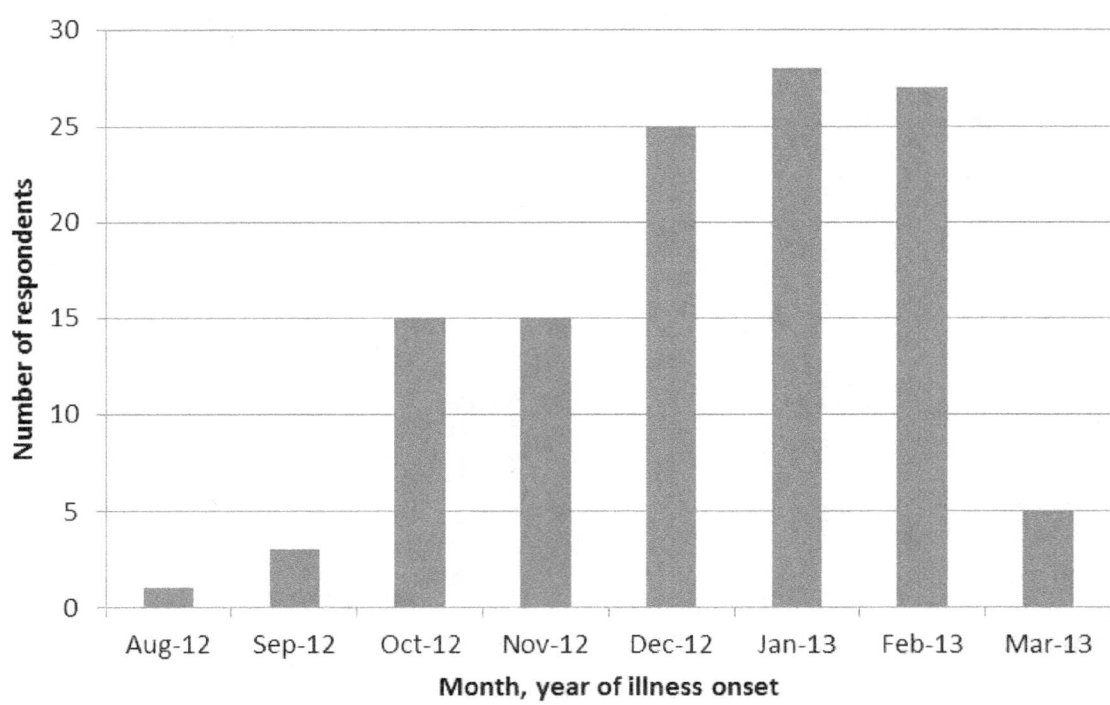

Figure 3. Month and year of onset of influenza-like illness symptoms among respondents.

The prevalence of reported ILI symptoms of the two most common groups was 30.4% for teachers and 28.8% for aides/paraprofessionals. The median days taken off work due to ILI was 1 day (range: 0–7 days). The total number of days taken off work was 162 days. A total of 92 (77%) of 120 respondents who reported ILI symptoms reported working while feeling sick. Eight reported working less than 1 day, 60 reported working 1–3 days, and 22 reported working 4 or more days. The two most common main reasons cited by respondents for working while ill were "I have a professional obligation to my students" (n = 25) and "I did not think I was contagious or could make other people sick" (n = 21). Other common main reasons are shown in Table 9.

Table 9. Main reasons cited by respondents for working while ill

Main reason cited*	No. (%) respondents n = 90
I have a professional obligation to my students.	25 (28)
I did not think I was contagious or could make other people sick.	21 (23)
It is difficult for me to get or prepare for a substitute.	11 (12)
I thought I might be penalized by my employer.	10 (11)
I have a professional obligation to my coworkers.	8 (9)
Other	15 (17)

*Respondents were asked to choose one main reason.

Regarding hand hygiene practices, 361 (88%) of 409 respondents reported having a sink with soap or alcohol-based hand sanitizer in their classroom or immediate work area. The median number of times respondents reported washing their hands with soap or using alcohol-based hand sanitizer during an average work day was 5 times (range: 0–30 times).

Respondents aged $\geq$ 50 years were 1.69 times more likely (95% CI = 1.07, 2.69) to have reported ILI symptoms than those aged < 50 years. We found no statistically significant associations between other demographic characteristics or work characteristics and reporting ILI symptoms. Regarding underlying medical conditions, those respondents with asthma were found to be 2.92 times more likely (95% CI = 1.20, 7.09) to have reported ILI symptoms than those without asthma. The other underlying medical conditions were not found to be significantly associated with reporting ILI symptoms. Reporting receipt of the influenza vaccine was not significantly associated with reporting ILI symptoms. In addition, having a sink with soap or alcohol-based sanitizer in the immediate work area and mean number of times of hand washing were not significantly associated with reporting ILI symptoms.

Discussion

Fifty-eight percent of responding school district employees reported having received the 2012–2013 influenza vaccine, despite the ACIP recommendation for annual influenza vaccination for all persons aged $\geq$ 6 months in the United States [CDC 2012d]. This vaccination coverage is similar to the one published study we found on school employees, in which Gargano and colleagues found that 62% of 66 surveyed school employees received the 2009–2010 seasonal influenza vaccine in two rural counties in Georgia [Gargano et al. 2011].

Influenza vaccination coverage among school employees in our survey (58%) is higher than that of the national estimates for the general U.S. adult population (39%) for the 2011–2012 influenza season [CDC 2013a]. It is also more than double the coverage seen in a population of child care workers (25%) for the 2009–2010 influenza season seen in the same county [de Perio et al. 2012]. In contrast, our findings are lower than the 2011–2012 influenza season coverage seen among U.S. healthcare personnel (67%). This difference is not surprising because healthcare personnel are considered a high risk occupational group and many efforts have focused on increasing vaccination coverage in this group [CDC 2012b].

We found that three major barriers to receiving the vaccine were that some school district employees did not believe they needed the vaccine, some did not think that the vaccine is effective, and some believed the vaccine would make them sick. These findings are similar to results from a national survey of healthcare personnel for the 2011–2012 influenza season [CDC 2012b] and multiple studies focusing on pandemic influenza vaccination among healthcare personnel [Prematunge et al. 2012]. Also, these reasons are similar to those most commonly cited by respondents of a community study examining intent to receive the 2009 pandemic influenza A (H1N1) vaccine [CDC 2009c]. Thus, these barriers are not exclusive to school employees and are present in healthcare personnel and the general population.

Another common main reason cited for not receiving the influenza vaccine was "I haven't had time to the get the flu vaccine." Our results show that the central district office was the most common place where respondents were vaccinated and that employees working out of the central district office were more likely to have received the influenza vaccine than those working in other locations. This suggests that providing vaccination at each of the schools may improve vaccination rates. In the United States during the 2010–2011 influenza vaccination season the workplace was the second most common vaccination location outside a doctor's office [CDC 2011c]. Annual workplace influenza vaccination reduces absenteeism and provides cost savings to employers [Nichol et al. 2003; Rothberg and Rose 2005; Prosser et al. 2008; Lee et al. 2010].

We found that respondents who reported receiving the 2011–2012 influenza vaccine more likely to have received the 2012–2013 influenza vaccine. Previous seasonal influenza vaccination has also been a commonly cited predictor of subsequent pandemic and seasonal influenza vaccination in studies of healthcare workers and the general adult population [Brien et al. 2012; Frew et al. 2012; Prematunge et al. 2012]. Therefore, changing an employee's negative beliefs about and attitudes towards the influenza vaccine has the potential to convert that employee to a yearly "adopter." Future vaccination campaigns should emphasize the necessity of yearly influenza vaccination.

Factors independently associated with receipt of the influenza vaccine included having beliefs that it is effective and safe, having positive attitudes toward the vaccine, feeling external pressure to get vaccinated, and feeling personal control over whether or not to get the vaccine. These findings suggest that employees' attitudes and beliefs about the influenza vaccine were more predictive of receipt of the vaccine than demographic and work characteristics and underlying medical conditions. These findings are similar to those of Gargano and colleagues, who determined that H1N1 vaccine uptake was associated with perceived barriers and social norms [Gargano et al. 2011]. Because perceiving pressure to get the vaccine was associated with receipt of the vaccine, physicians, employers, unions, teachers' associations, health insurers, and school boards should improve efforts to recommend influenza vaccination for school employees.

Being classified as obese or reporting an underlying medical condition associated with high risk of serious influenza-related complications, including diabetes; asthma; kidney, heart, and liver disease; cancer; and immunosuppressive conditions, was not significantly associated with receipt of the vaccine. Though the percentage of respondents who reported these conditions was low, this finding suggests that public health messages targeting vaccine promotion in these high risk groups may have been ineffective, and that efforts to improve coverage in this population should be strengthened. Those sources mentioned above could be valuable in providing these health messages.

Almost one third of our respondents reported ILI during the school year, with a peak occurring in January 2013. To our knowledge, this is the first evaluation to determine prevalence of ILI among school employees. We found that respondents aged ≥ 50 years and those with asthma, both known risk factors for influenza complications [CDC 2010b; CDC 2012c], were more likely to have reported ILI symptoms. Though we did not find a significant association between reporting ILI symptoms and reporting receipt of the influenza vaccine, this survey was not designed to determine the effectiveness of the influenza vaccine. Our analysis was limited in that we could not determine if the cause of ILI symptoms was from influenza infection or another virus or a bacterial infection.

We also found that 77% of those respondents with ILI reported working while feeling sick, suggesting that presenteeism (i.e., attending work while ill) is quite common in this school district. Presenteeism leads to decreased productivity but also leads to the potential for transmission of infectious diseases in the workplace [Widera et al. 2010]. Our findings are similar to a survey that found that nearly 83% of participants from the U.S. population reported continuing to attend work or school while experiencing ILI symptoms [CDC 2004]. Ablah and colleagues found that 57% of school system employees in one county in Kansas reported having worked with an ILI [Ablah et al. 2008].

The two most common reasons cited by respondents for working while ill were "I have a professional obligation to my students" and "I did not think I was contagious or could make other people sick." Thus, targeting messaging to school employees that addresses these barriers may benefit the school district in the future. District policies should also ensure adequate staffing and coverage of employees to limit feelings of personal responsibility that encourage presenteeism.

Our evaluation was subject to some limitations. First, respondents self-reported their receipt of the vaccine and ILI symptoms, and this may have been subject to recall errors. Vaccination was not validated by medical records. Second, our evaluation focused on employees of one suburban school district in Ohio, and our results may not be generalizable to employees in districts in urban and rural settings and in districts with more racial diversity. Third, our participation rate was 49%, despite multiple e-mail reminders from employer and teachers' association representatives. We believe several factors may have contributed to this less than optimal response rate. Because of initial technical difficulties, the Web survey was inaccessible over periods of time. Also, we did not have direct contact with all employees but relied on employer and teachers' association representatives to disseminate the survey for us. This less than optimal response rate raises the possibility that our results are not representative of all district employees, especially the operational employees, whose response rates (12%–22%) were lower than those of the educational employees (55%–61%). The response rate to our survey is actually higher than those seen in other electronic surveys (mean response rates between 19% and 40%), but lower rates are seen in larger surveys, workplace surveys, and surveys not offering incentives [Jones and Pitt 1999; Cook et al. 2000; Sheehan 2001; Manfreda and Vehovar 2002; Kaplowitz et al. 2004; Shih and Fan 2008]. Nevertheless, it is possible that our survey was subject to selection bias, and that we may have overestimated or underestimated the influenza vaccination rate among district employees.

Conclusions

Vaccination is the most effective method to prevent influenza and to prevent serious illness and death from influenza infection. Influenza vaccination coverage among the 49% responding school district employees was 58%. Factors independently associated with vaccine receipt were having positive attitudes toward the vaccine, feeling external pressure to get vaccinated, and feeling personal control over whether or not to get the vaccine. Misconceptions about the need for the vaccine and its efficacy and the perception of not having enough time to get it were the most common reasons cited for not getting it. We also found that prevalence of ILI symptoms among respondents was 29%, and many reported working while ill. Our findings highlight the need to emphasize the benefits, safety, and effectiveness of vaccination and the importance of staying home when ill with ILI symptoms.

Recommendations

A comprehensive strategy to prevent the spread of influenza in the school district should include all of the following: vaccination of students, faculty, and staff; hand hygiene; respiratory etiquette; observing students for symptoms of respiratory illness; and encouraging sick students and employees to stay home. Vaccination is a pivotal part of this comprehensive strategy and is the most effective method to prevent serious illness and death from influenza infection [Cox and Subbarao 1999; Nichol and Treanor 2006]. Vaccination has been shown to reduce illness and absenteeism caused by influenza. School district employees should receive influenza vaccination to protect themselves, their families, and their students from influenza. Annual influenza vaccination is recommended for all persons aged ≥ 6 months who do not have contraindications to vaccination [CDC 2012d].

More comprehensive recommendations for influenza prevention can be found in CDC's Guidance for School Administrators to Help Reduce the Spread of Seasonal Influenza in K–12 Schools at http://www.cdc.gov/flu/school/guidance.htm.

The three key phases to a successful vaccination campaign are notification, education, and vaccination [Hofmann et al. 2006]. On the basis of our findings, we recommend actions corresponding to these key phases and list them below to increase influenza vaccination rates among employees in the school district.

Recommendations for the School District, Unions, and Teachers' Association

1. Recommend the influenza vaccine to all employees.

2. Encourage employees to get vaccinated by including messages in e-mails, posters throughout work locations, staff newsletters, and staff meetings. Messages should be encouraging and highlight motivators for employees such as protecting themselves, family members, and the students with whom they interact. Suggested messages are "To protect the health of our students, as well as yourself and your family, it's

recommended that you get a flu shot," and "Our students and families thank you for helping to keep the flu out of [school name]. Get vaccinated!" or "Protect yourself, your family, and your students from the flu by getting vaccinated!" Messages can also address the most frequent antivaccination ideas, including the perceived low risk for infection, perceived lack of vaccine efficacy, and lack of knowledge of vaccine safety.

3. Develop a committee with employer, union, teachers' association, and other employee representation to explore the feasibility of offering annual influenza vaccination to employees at each school, the transportation department, and the maintenance building. Continue partnering with local vaccine providers to offer the vaccine to employees at no or low cost. Obtain up-to-date information on pharmacy locations that offer the influenza vaccine, encourage employees to obtain it, and share the information with them through e-mail, newsletters, or informational sheets.

4. Emphasize the importance of influenza vaccination among pregnant women and individuals with high-risk medical conditions in health messages. These groups are at highest risk for developing influenza-related complications [CDC 2012c].

5. Identify an employee or employees (members and non-members of the unions and teachers' association) with previous influenza vaccination history who can advocate for the receipt of the influenza vaccine to coworkers. Provide this employee "champion" with information regarding the benefits of influenza vaccination, and encourage this employee to share this information throughout the workplace. This approach has been shown to be effective in increasing influenza vaccination rates among healthcare personnel [Slaunwhite et al. 2009].

6. Consider offering incentives to employees who get vaccinated. Suggestions include raffles of gift cards. Creating friendly competition among schools to achieve the highest rates can be considered; the winner could be rewarded with a prize such as a free lunch.

7. Develop a committee with employer, union, teachers' association, and other employee representation to explore creating a policy requiring employees to get the influenza vaccine as part of a comprehensive influenza prevention strategy. Implementing this requirement has been demonstrated to be effective among healthcare personnel [CDC 2010b].

8. Encourage employees to self-assess for ILI symptoms and to stay home when sick according to CDC guidance at http://www.cdc.gov/flu/school/guidance.htm. Employees should stay home when sick until at least 24 hours after they no longer have a fever (100° Fahrenheit or 37.8° Celsius) or signs of a fever (chills, feeling very warm, flushed appearance, or sweating) without the use of fever-reducing medicine. Review school policies, and consider revising those that make it difficult for employees to stay home when sick. Avoid using perfect attendance awards.

9. Encourage hand hygiene among employees and students through education, scheduled time for hand washing, and the provision of supplies. Teach students and staff to wash hands often with soap and water for 20 seconds, dry hands with a paper towel, and use the paper towel to turn off the faucet. If soap and water are not available and hands are

not visibly dirty, an alcohol-based hand sanitizer containing at least 60% alcohol may be used. Additional information on hand hygiene can be found at http://www.cdc.gov/handwashing/, CDC's basic hand hygiene website, and at http://www.itsasnap.org/snap/about.asp, which contains school-specific information.

Recommendations for School District Employees

1. Get the seasonal influenza vaccine every year. Additional vaccination locations other than those offered at the school district are available on the county public health department flu shot location website at http://www.hamiltoncountyhealth.org/resourceSearch.aspx?publish=1&lang=en&type=4 or by calling (513) 931-SHOT. Additional information for flu shot providers nationwide can be found at http://www.flucliniclocator.org/.

2. Stay informed. Obtain information about influenza and the influenza vaccine from reliable sources. The National Library of Medicine and the National Institutes of Health offer guidelines for evaluating the quality of health information at http://www.nlm.nih.gov/medlineplus/evaluatinghealthinformation.html.

3. Discuss other options for preventing influenza with your healthcare provider if you have any contraindications to receiving either the influenza injection or nasal vaccine.

4. Be an influenza vaccine "champion," and encourage your coworkers to get the influenza vaccine.

5. Self-assess for symptoms of ILI. Report any symptoms to appropriate supervisors as soon as possible. Do not report for work when ill according to CDC guidance at http://www.cdc.gov/flu/school/guidance.htm.

6. Obtain more information on other ways to protect yourself and prevent the spread of influenza in schools at http://www.cdc.gov/flu/school/.

References

Ablah E, Konda K, Tinius A, Long R, Vermie G, Burbach C [2008]. Influenza vaccine coverage and presenteeism in Sedgwick County, Kansas. Am J Infect Control 36(8):588–591.

Adams PF, Hendershot GE, Marano MA [1999]. Current estimates from the National Health Interview Survey, 1996. Vital Health Stat 10(200):1–203.

Ajzen I [1991]. The theory of planned behavior. Organ Behav Hum Decis Process 50(2):179–211.

Armitage CJ, Conner M [2001]. Efficacy of the theory of planned behaviour: a metaanalytic review. Br J Soc Psychol 40(Pt 4):471–499.

Blachere FM, Lindsley WG, Pearce TA, Anderson SE, Fisher M, Khakoo R, Meade BJ, Lander O, Davis S, Thewlis RE, Celik I, Chen BT, Beezhold DH [2009]. Measurement of airborne influenza virus in a hospital emergency department. Clin Infect Dis 48(15):438–440.

Bridges CB, Thompson WW, Martin MI, Reeve GR, Talamonti WJ, Cox NJ, Lilac HA, Hall H, Klimov A, Fujuda K [2000]. Effectiveness and cost-benefit of influenza vaccination of health working adults: a randomized controlled trial. JAMA 284(13):1655–1663.

Bridges CB, Kuehnert MJ, Hall CB [2003]. Transmission of influenza: implications for control in health care settings. Clin Infect Dis 37(8):1094–1101.

Brien S, Kwong JC, Buckeridge DL [2012]. The determinants of 2009 pandemic A/H1N1 influenza vaccination: a systematic review. Vaccine 30(7):1255–1264.

CDC (Centers for Disease Control and Prevention) [2004]. Experiences with influenza-like illness and attitudes regarding influenza prevention — United States, 2003–04 influenza season. MMWR 53(49):1156–1158.

CDC (Centers for Disease Control and Prevention) [2009a]. National 2009 H1N1 flu survey questionnaire. Atlanta, Georgia: U.S. Department of Health and Human Services, Centers for Disease Control and Prevention.

CDC (Centers for Disease Control and Prevention) [2009b]. Intensive-care patients with severe novel influenza A (H1N1) virus infection — Michigan, June 2009. MMWR 58(27):749–752.

CDC (Centers for Disease Control and Prevention) [2009c]. Intent to receive influenza A (H1N1) 2009 monovalent and seasonal influenza vaccines — Two counties, North Carolina, August 2009. MMWR 58(50):1401–1404.

CDC (Centers for Disease Control and Prevention) [2010a]. Estimates of deaths associated with seasonal influenza — United States, 1976–2007. MMWR 59(33):1057–1062.

CDC (Centers for Disease Control and Prevention) [2010b]. Prevention and control of influenza with vaccines: recommendations of the Advisory Committee on Immunization Practices (ACIP). MMWR *59*(No. RR-8):1–62.

CDC (Centers for Disease Control and Prevention) [2011a]. Behavioral risk factor surveillance system survey questionnaire. Atlanta, Georgia: U.S. Department of Health and Human Services, Centers for Disease Control and Prevention. [http://www.cdc.gov/brfss/questionnaires/pdf-ques/2011brfss.pdf]. Date accessed: July 2013.

CDC (Centers for Disease Control and Prevention) [2011b]. Body mass index. [http://www.cdc.gov/healthyweight/assessing/bmi/index.html]. Date accessed: July 2013.

CDC (Centers for Disease Control and Prevention) [2011c]. Place of influenza vaccination among adults — United States, 2010–11 influenza season. MMWR *60*(23):781–785.

CDC (Centers for Disease Control and Prevention) [2012a]. Guidance for school administrators to help reduce the spread of seasonal influenza in K–12 schools. [http://www.cdc.gov/flu/school/guidance.htm]. Date accessed: July 2013.

CDC (Centers for Disease Control and Prevention) [2012b]. Influenza vaccination coverage among health-care personnel: 2011–12 influenza season, United States. MMWR *61*(38):753–757.

CDC (Centers for Disease Control and Prevention) [2012c]. Key facts about influenza (flu) & flu vaccine. [http://www.cdc.gov/flu/keyfacts.htm]. Date accessed: July 2013.

CDC (Centers for Disease Control and Prevention) [2012d]. Prevention and control of influenza with vaccines: recommendations of the Advisory Committee on Immunization Practices (ACIP) — United States, 2012–13 influenza season. MMWR *61*(32):613–618.

CDC (Centers for Disease Control and Prevention) [2013a]. Flu vaccination coverage, United States, 2011–12 Influenza Season. [http://www.cdc.gov/flu/professionals/vaccination/coverage_1112estimates.htm]. Date accessed: July 2013.

CDC (Centers for Disease Control and Prevention) [2013b]. Interim adjusted estimates of seasonal influenza vaccine effectiveness — United States, February 2013. MMWR *62*(7):119–123.

Cook C, Heath F, Thompson RL [2000]. A meta-analysis of response rates in Web- or Internet-based surveys. Educ Psychol Meas *60*(6):821–836.

Cox NJ, Subbarao K [1999]. Influenza. Lancet *354*(9186):1277–1282.

de Perio MA, Wiegand DM, Evans SM [2012]. Low influenza vaccination rates among child care workers in the United States: assessing knowledge, attitudes, and behaviors. J Comm Health *37*(2):272–281.

Francis JJ, Eccles MP, Johnston M, Walker A, Grimshaw J, Foy R. Kaner EFS, Zmith L, Bonetti D [2004]. Constructing questionnaires based on the theory of planned behavior: a manual for health services researchers. University of Newcastle Upon Tyne: Centre for Health Services Research edition. University of Newcastle Upon Tyne.

Frew PM, Painter JE, Fixson B, Kulb C, Moore K, del Rio C, Esteves-Jaramillo A, Omer SB [2012]. Factors mediating seasonal and influenza A (H1N1) vaccine acceptance among ethnically diverse populations in the urban south. Vaccine *30*(28):4200–4208.

Fukuda K, Levandowski RA, Bridges CB, Cox NJ [2004]. Inactivated influenza vaccines. In: Plotkin SA, Orenstein WA, eds. Vaccines. 4th ed. Philadelphia, PA: Saunders, pp. 339–370.

Gargano LM, Painter JE, Sales JM, Morfaw C, Jones LM, Murray D, Wingood GM, DiClemente RJ, Hughes JM [2011]. Seasonal and 2009 H1N1 influenza vaccine uptake, predictors of vaccination, and self-reported barriers to vaccination among secondary school teachers and staff. Hum Vaccin *7*(1):89–95.

Hofmann F, Ferracin C, Marsh, G, Dumas R [2006]. Influenza vaccination of healthcare workers: a literature review of attitudes and beliefs. Infection *34*(3):142–147.

Jain S, Kamimoto L, Bramley AM, Schmitz AM, Benoit SR, Louie J, Sugerman DE, Druckenmiller JK, Ritger KA, Chugh R, Jasuja S, Deutscher M, Chen S, Walker JD, Duchin JS, Lett S, Soliva S, Wells EV, Swerdlow D, Uyeki TM, Fiore AE, Olsen SJ, Fry AM, Bridges CB, Finelli L; 2009 Pandemic Influenza A (H1N1) Virus Hospitalizations Investigation Team [2009]. Hospitalized patients with 2009 H1N1 influenza in the United States, April–June 2009. N Engl J Med *361*(20):1935–1944.

Jones R, Pitt N [1999]. Health surveys in the workplace: comparison of postal, email, and World Wide Web methods. Occup Med *49*(8):556–558.

Kaplowitz MD, Hadlock TD, Levine R [2004]. A comparison of web and mail survey response rates. Public Opin Q *68*(1):94–101.

Kumar A, Zarychanski R, Pinto R, Cook DJ, Marshall J, Lacroix J, Stelfox T, Bagshaw S, Choong K, Lamontagne F, Turgeon AF, Lapinsky S, Ahern SP, Smith O, Siddiqui F, Jouvet P, Khwaja K, McIntyre L, Menon K, Hutchison J, Hornstein D, Joffe A, Lauzier F, Singh J, Karachi T, Wiebe K, Olafson K, Ramsey C, Sharma S, Dodek P, Meade M, Hall R, Fowler RA; Canadian Critical Care Trials Group H1N1 Collaborative [2009]. Critically ill patients with 2009 influenza A(H1N1) infection in Canada. JAMA *302*(17):1872–1879.

Kwong JC, Campitelli MA, Rosella LC [2011]. Obesity and respiratory hospitalizations during influenza seasons in Ontario, Canada, a cohort study. Clin Infect Dis *53*(5):413–421.

Lee BY, Bailey RR, Wiringa AE, Afriyie A, Wateska AR, Smith KJ, Zimmerman RK [2010]. Economics of employer-sponsored workplace vaccination to prevent pandemic and seasonal influenza. Vaccine *28*(37):5952–5959.

Lindsley WG, Blachere FM, Davis KA, Pearce TA, Fisher MA, Khakoo R, Davis SM,. Rogers ME, Thewlis RE, Posada JA, Redrow JB, Celik IB, Chen BT, Beezhold DH [2010a]. Distribution of airborne influenza virus and respiratory syncytial virus in an urgent care medical clinic. Clin Infect Dis *50*(5):693–698.

Lindsley WG, Blachere FM, Thewlis RE, Vishnu A, Davis KA, Cao G, Palmer JE, Clark KE, Fisher MA, Khakoo R, Beezhold DH [2010b]. Measurements of airborne influenza virus in aerosol particles from human coughs. PLoS One *5*(11):e15100.

Louie JK, Acosta M, Winter K, Jean C, Gavali S, Schechter R, Vugia D, Harriman K, Matyas B, Glaser CA, Samuel MC, Rosenberg J, Talarico J, Hatch D; California Pandemic (H1N1) Working Group [2009]. Factors associated with death or hospitalization due to pandemic 2009 influenza A(H1N1) infection in California. JAMA *302*(17):1896–1902.

Manfreda KL, Vehovar V [2002]. Survey design features influencing response rates in Web surveys. University of Copenhagen, Denmark: The International Conference on Improving Surveys. [http://www.websm.org/uploadi/editor/Lozar_Vehovar_2001_Survey_design.pdf]. Date accessed: July 2013.

Molinari NA, Ortega-Sanchez IR, Messonnier ML, Thompson WW, Wortley PM, Weintraub E, Bridges CB [2007]. The annual impact of seasonal influenza in the U.S.: measuring disease burden and costs. Vaccine *25*(27):5086–5096.

Nichol KL, Treanor JJ [2006]. Vaccines for seasonal and pandemic influenza. J Infect Dis *194*(Suppl2):S111–118.

Nichol KL, Lind A, Margolis KL, Murdoc M, McFadden R, Hauge M, Magnan S, Drake M [1995]. The effectiveness of vaccination against influenza in healthy, working adults. N Engl J Med *333*(14):889–893.

Nichol KL, Mallon KP, Mendelman PM [2003]. Cost benefit of influenza vaccination in healthy, working adults: an economic analysis based on the results of a clinical trial of trivalent live attenuated influenza virus vaccine. Vaccine *21*(17–18):2207–2217.

Pedhazur EJ [1997]. Multiple regression in behavioral research: explanation and prediction. 3rd ed. New York: Thompson Learning, Inc.

Prematunge C, Corace K, McCarthy A, Nair RC, Pugsley R, Garber G [2012]. Factors influencing pandemic influenza vaccination of healthcare workers – a systematic review. Vaccine *30*(32):4733–4743.

Prosser LA, O'Brien MA, Molinari NA, Hohman KH, Nichol KL, Messonnier ML, Lieu T [2008]. Non-traditional settings for influenza vaccination of adults: costs and cost effectiveness. Pharmacoecon *26*(2):163–178.

Rothberg MB, Rose DN [2005]. Vaccination versus treatment of influenza in working adults: a cost-effectiveness analysis. Am J Med *118*(1):68–77.

Sheehan K [2001]. E-mail survey response rates: a review. J Comput Mediat Commun *16*(2). [http://jcmc.indiana.edu/vol6/issue2/sheehan.html]. Date accessed: July 2013.

Shih T-H, Fan X [2008]. Comparing response rates from Web and mail surveys: a meta-analysis. Field Methods *20*(3):249–271.

Slaunwhite JM, Smith SM, Fleming MT [2009]. Increasing vaccination rates among health care workers using unit "champions" as a motivator. Can J Infect Control *24*(3):159–164.

Thompson WW, Shay DK, Weintraub E, Brammer L, Cox NJ, Fukuda K [2004]. Influenza-associated hospitalizations in the United States. JAMA *292*(11):1333–1340.

U.S. Department of Health and Human Services [2013]. Immunization and infectious diseases. [http://www.healthypeople.gov/2020/topicsobjectives2020/objectiveslist.aspx?topicId=23]. Date accessed: July 2013.

Vellozzi C, Burwen DR, Dobardzic A, Ball R, Walton K, Haber P [2009]. Safety of trivalent inactivated influenza vaccines in adults: background for pandemic influenza vaccine safety monitoring. Vaccine *27*(15):2114–2120.

Widera E, Chang A, Chen HL [2010]. Presenteeism: a public health hazard. J Gen Intern Med *25*(11):1244–1247.

Wright PF, Webster RG [2001]. Orthomyxoviruses. In: Knipe DM, Howley PM, eds. Fields virology. 4th ed. Philadelphia, PA: Lippincott Williams & Wilkins, pp. 1534–1579.

Keywords: North American Industry Classification System 611110 (Elementary and Secondary Schools), influenza, vaccination, immunization, school, teachers, infection

The Health Hazard Evaluation Program investigates possible health hazards in the workplace under the authority of Section 20(a)(6) of the Occupational Safety and Health Act of 1970, 29 U.S.C. 669(a)(6). The Health Hazard Evaluation Program also provides, upon request, technical assistance to federal, state, and local agencies to control occupational health hazards and to prevent occupational illness and disease. Regulations guiding the Program can be found in Title 42, Code of Federal Regulations, Part 85; Requests for Health Hazard Evaluations (42 CFR 85).

Acknowledgments

Desktop Publisher: Mary Winfree
Editor: Ellen Galloway
Health Communicator: Stefanie Brown
Technical Support: David Nitschke, Harold Collins, and Mohammad Islam, CDC/OSELS; MeeHee Cho, University of Cincinnati
Subject Matter Consultation: Stacie Greby and Tara Vogt, CDC/NCIRD

Availability of Report

Copies of this report have been sent to the employer and employees at the installation. The state and local health department and the Occupational Safety and Health Administration Regional Office have also received a copy. This report is not copyrighted and may be freely reproduced.

This report is available at http://www.cdc.gov/niosh/hhe/reports/pdfs/2013-0064-3191.pdf.

Recommended citation for this report:
NIOSH [2013]. Health hazard evaluation report: evaluation of knowledge, attitudes, and practices regarding influenza vaccination among employees in a school district. By de Perio MA, Wiegand DM, Brueck SE. Cincinnati, OH: U.S. Department of Health and Human Services, Centers for Disease Control and Prevention, National Institute for Occupational Safety and Health, NIOSH HHE Report No. 2013-0064-3191.